CHARLES WEAVER

No longer fearing Alzheimer's Disease

The layman's guide to avoiding and reversing Alzheimer-type dementia

Copyright © 2024 by Charles Weaver

All rights reserved. No part of this publication may be reproduced, stored or transmitted in any form or by any means, electronic, mechanical, photocopying, recording, scanning, or otherwise without written permission from the publisher. It is illegal to copy this book, post it to a website, or distribute it by any other means without permission.

Charles Weaver asserts the moral right to be identified as the author of this work.

Charles Weaver has no responsibility for the persistence or accuracy of URLs for external or third-party Internet Websites referred to in this publication and does not guarantee that any content on such Websites is, or will remain, accurate or appropriate.

Designations used by companies to distinguish their products are often claimed as trademarks. All brand names and product names used in this book and on its cover are trade names, service marks, trademarks and registered trademarks of their respective owners. The publishers and the book are not associated with any product or vendor mentioned in this book. None of the companies referenced within the book have endorsed the book.

First edition

This book was professionally typeset on Reedsy.
Find out more at reedsy.com

Contents

1	Introduction	1
2	What exactly is Alzheimer's Disease?	4
3	Research directions and who decided that these were the best...	8
4	The 'one root cause' phenomenon ...	12
5	Why pharmaceuticals are an unlikely successful...	16
6	Prevention and Recovery	18
7	You must understand that lifestyle choices are paramount	22
8	Identifying toxins and removing their sources	25
9	Mindset	30
10	Conclusions	32
11	Resources	33

1

Introduction

Welcome to the No Longer Fearing Alzheimer's Disease manual. My name is Charles Weaver, PhD. For the longest time, my family members and friends have worried endlessly about the possibilities of developing Alzheimer's Disease (AD). I'm here to tell you that the medical and scientific communities have made tremendous strides into elucidating both the risk factors and treatments for AD. Yes, there are books available that will explain these in greater depths; but honestly, most people want the crib sheet. Well, here it is.

As someone who has studied AD since the early 1990s, it is my pleasure to share this information with you. People should enjoy their lives to the fullest extent. However, the conveniences of modern-day life have contributed mightily to this dreaded disease. It's time we address this clearly and succinctly.

Let me share a little bit of background information about me. I have a PhD in Neuroscience and have spent most of my time researching topics such as brain infection and neurodegeneration, human variations in biochemistry, and the effects of earth's frequencies on health. I've split time between academia and some of the poorest countries in the world. This has afforded me the opportunity to affirm the etiologies of chronic disease, most being rooted in modern-day lifestyles and exposure to environmental toxins. Personally, I've incorporated several strategies to maintain my health as I age by simplifying my life. These are not difficult although many are costly. I hope to express their benefit in this book.

While there is a chance that you will not utilize these strategies to their fullest extent, I maintain that they are worthwhile in easing your fears about the development of Alzheimer's Disease. No one wants to lose the autonomy of adulthood. When you think about AD, visualize your loved one reverting from an adult to a child. This is what happens. Not only will they become completely dependent upon your assistance, they may also develop primitive reflexes and associated movements. You see, losing your short-term memory is just a small part of the pathology. I understand that having a loved one forget your name is daunting enough. But it's crucial that you embrace the realities of the entire situation, without becoming overwhelmed. Again, there are strategies for preventing and overcoming AD. This brief read is meant to encourage you to get there in the shortest time while acknowledging the incredible work done by scientists and clinicians.

If there is even the slightest amount of apprehension about the realities of what is shared in this book, please don't worry. You are free to read other intensive and in-depth books on this topic.

INTRODUCTION

However, time is short. Decades seem to fly by because of all the busyness that society has thrusted upon us. Let's get to the truth right now. You and your loved ones will be grateful that you did. In a healthy society, people have an interest not only for themselves, but for their community (family, friends, others), as well. Let's restore health...and do it the right way!

2

What exactly is Alzheimer's Disease?

Aloysius Alzheimer - the man who started it all...or did he?

Alzheimer's Disease (AD) is named after prominent clinician Aloysius Alzheimer. He deftly described a case first encountered in March of 1901 where Auguste Deter was brought by her husband to the Psychiatric Hospital at Frankfurt because of bouts of confusion, sleep disturbances, and memory loss. He followed this case closely over the next 4+ years until her death in April of 1906. In November of 1906, Alzheimer presented his clinical findings, along with an initial neuropathology report, at a psychiatric meeting in Tubingen, Germany. The talk received little attention from many prominent scientists and later was described by only a very brief abstract.[1]

After moving to Munich in 1903, and around the time of Deter's death in 1906, Alzheimer was also promoted to deputy director at the Psychiatric University Hospital. Because of the significant increase in responsibilities, Alzheimer entrusted Gaetano

Perusini to conduct detailed histopathological findings of Deter and three other cases.[1] Perusini, exceptionally skilled in the visualization and determination of senile plaques and neurofibrillary tangles associated with senile dementia, expertly described the progression of these pathologies within the aforementioned cases.[2,3] This report was published in 1909.

Ultimately, Emil Kraepelin, contemporary and coworker of Aloysius, coined the diagnosis of Alzheimer's disease in 1910. In a sense, Alzheimer was the first to experience this case, while Perusini was instrumental in the detailed description of its pathologies.

Should the disease be named differently? That may be a stretch. What's more important is that something happened around that time which contributed to the emergence of the disease. What was it? Can it/they be classified as one thing? Well see in a subsequent chapter. Nevertheless, by understanding the factors contributing to the disease, we can begin to understand the need for a multitude of specific therapeutics.

Classic neuropathological hallmarks

While the neuropathological hallmarks of Alzheimer's Disease are numerous and varied, ranging from amyloid plaques, to tangles, to tau hyperphosphorylation, to cerebral amyloid angiopathy, and glial disturbances, the two most prominent hallmarks are the beta-amyloid plaque and the neurofibrillary tangle.

Defining 'hallmark'

The word 'hallmark' simply means to say officially that something is distinctive. There you have it. Nothing more. It does not mean that something is causative. Herein is the problem with research. For too long, science has looked at hallmarks and pursued their course. When this stance is immediately taken, it often takes decades to reverse action and investigate something more relevant. Such is the case with Alzheimer Disease.

Amyloid plaques – diffuse vs neuritic

The amyloid protein begins as a transmembrane (i.e., embedded into the cell membrane) structure called the amyloid precursor protein (APP).[5] It plays many roles in the body; but in the brain, it is involved in cell-to-cell communication via its interaction with a structure known as the synapse (junction). It generally has two pathways of processing: 1) synapse-enhancing or 2) synapse-destroying. In Alzheimer's Disease, the APP molecule is cleaved into a smaller component called beta-amyloid.[6] Beta-amyloid aggregates and disrupts synaptic integrity.

Diffuse plaques are usually loosely bound together beta-amyloid fragments.[7] They often have wool or cotton-like appearances and can be seen in pathological and non-pathological settings. Neuritic plaques are beta-amyloid aggregates that have a compact or dense core. The neuritic elements are swollen axons, or sometimes dendrites. The vast majority of neuritic plaques are found in the later stages of AD.[8]

Neurofibrillary tangles

The second notable neuropathological hallmark is known as the neurofibrillary tangle (NFT). NFTs are generated by aggregation of the tau protein which has been modified by the addition of many phosphate groups (i.e., hyperphosphorylation).[9] Hyperphosphorylated tau aggregates begin as subset structures known as paired helical filaments (PHFs) and then clump into larger NFT masses.[10]

Neurofibrillary tangles are an early phenomenon in AD. Their presence has been significantly correlated with the onset and severity of dementia. Being intracellular in nature, it is easy to see how they can be involved in neuronal destruction. However, loss of neurons often occurs before the presence of NFTs.[11]

Others

As noted, the two classic neuropathological hallmarks are plaques and tangles. Cerebral amyloid angiopathy generally occurs later in the cascade of events and glial disturbances are yet to be elucidated as early factors involved in neuronal loss.

3

Research directions and who decided that these were the best approaches, anyway?

early 1900s, infection

Some of Aloysius Alzheimer's early work centered around syphilis.[12] Many patients exhibiting disrupted mental status had syphilis, prompting Alzheimer to loosely speculate on the role of infection in brain degeneration. Ironically, Alzheimer would rule out nutritional disorders as a basis of dementia.[12] Perhaps, this set the field spiraling in the wrong direction for decades as this manual will acknowledge how the current understanding of nutrition highlights its significant role in the etiology of AD. Nevertheless, infection does generate a substantial amount of inflammation in the Alzheimer brain.[13] This, most certainly, leads to both the loss of synapses and destruction of neurons.

1950 - 1980, neurotransmitters & brain chemistry, heavy metals,

and lipids

Much of the research during this time included analyses of neurotransmitters. In Alzheimer's Disease, neurotransmitters were thought to play a crucial role, primarily because the disease affects communication among neurons in the brain. Neurotransmitters are chemicals that transmit signals between neurons. These signals are essential for various brain functions, including memory, learning, and cognition. One of the key neurotransmitters affected in AD is acetylcholine. Acetylcholine is involved in memory and learning processes. In Alzheimer's, there is a significant reduction in the levels of acetylcholine due to the loss of cholinergic neurons in the brain. This loss of acetylcholine, at the time, was thought to significantly contribute to the memory deficits and cognitive decline seen in Alzheimer's patients.[14]

Additionally, other neurotransmitter systems are also affected in Alzheimer's Disease, including glutamate, serotonin, and dopamine. Imbalances in these neurotransmitters can further contribute to the cognitive and behavioral symptoms of Alzheimer's.[14]

The role of heavy metals in Alzheimer's Disease was just gathering steam and began generating much debate in the scientific community. A number of studies suggested that exposure to certain heavy metals may be associated with an increased risk of developing Alzheimer's Disease or exacerbating its symptoms.[15]

Heavy metals such as aluminum, lead, cadmium, and mercury have been found to accumulate in the brain over time, particularly in regions affected by Alzheimer's disease. Heavy metals can also induce oxidative stress and trigger neurotoxicity, leading to damage to neurons and potentially contributing to the progression of Alzheimer's Disease.[15] Some research suggested that certain heavy metals may promote the aggregation and accumulation of beta-amyloid proteins and neurofibrillary tangles, both of which are hallmarks of AD pathology.[16] Lastly, heavy metal exposure were shown to trigger inflammatory responses and dysregulate the immune system, which may further contribute to neurodegeneration and Alzheimer's disease progression.[15]

Lipids, which include fats and fat-like substances such as cholesterol, were explored in earnest simply because neuronal cell membranes are made of them. The composition and properties of these membranes, such as fluidity, influence the function of membrane-associated proteins (think beta-amyloid) and are involved in signaling, synaptic plasticity, and neuronal communication—all of which are impaired in Alzheimer's Disease.[17]

1980 - 2000, enter nutrition

Perhaps being annoyed with a lack of a cause, researchers began studying the role of nutrition in brain chemistry. While the role of nutrition was in its infancy, clear steps began to emerge. Micronutrients, or the lack thereof, played a role in the cognitive health of patients.[18] These nutrients were in the form of vitamins and minerals. Also, certain fats seemed to decrease the risk of cognitive impairment while others increased it.[18] The gut-brain axis and its role in the generation of inflammation and reduced immune responses[18] seemed to propel research into new ideas on Alzheimer etiology. These branches of research would ultimately prove efficacious in not only demonstrating how nutrition could affect the generation of plaques and tangles, but also the generation of treatment protocols.

Who decided...???

This begs the question, "Who decided that nutrition was unimportant?" OK, let's not jump on the 'Big Pharma did it' bandwagon just yet. From what we've previously read, we may just have to point the finger at Aloysius Alzheimer.

4

The 'one root cause' phenomenon and why there isn't such a thing

Have you ever heard that researchers are looking for 'the cause' of a certain neurodegenerative disease? If this is a reality in Alzheimer's Disease, then why haven't these brilliant scientists and clinicians been able to figure this out in over 100 years? The simplest explanation is that there isn't such a thing...i.e., there isn't one cause. Let's explore.

The magic bullet and modern-day snake oil salesmen

Currently, there are two main classes of drugs approved for the treatment of Alzheimer's Disease: cholinesterase inhibitors and NMDA receptor agonists.

Cholinesterase inhibitors work by increasing levels of acetylcholine, a neurotransmitter involved in memory and learning, by inhibiting the enzyme that breaks it down (acetylcholinesterase).[19] By doing so, they help improve cognitive symptoms in some people with Alzheimer's Disease. The three cholinesterase inhibitors approved by the U.S. Food and Drug Administration (FDA) for the treatment of AD are:

- Donepezil (brand name: Aricept)
- Rivastigmine (brand names: Exelon, Exelon Patch)
- Galantamine (brand names: Razadyne, Razadyne ER)

NMDA Receptor antagonists work by regulating glutamate, another neurotransmitter involved in learning and memory. NMDA receptor antagonists block the action of excess glutamate, which can be toxic to neurons (cytotoxic) in AD.[19] The NMDA receptor antagonist approved for Alzheimer's Disease treatment is:

- Memantine (brand names: Namenda, Namenda XR)

These medications may provide temporary symptomatic relief and may briefly help slow the progression of cognitive decline in some individuals with Alzheimer's Disease. However, it's important to note that they work only 6-12 months before causing side effects such as serious liver and kidney dysfunction.

So, here we are. There are two approved treatments in 100+ years of diligent research. Neither of these reverses cognitive decline. And to make matters worse, the side effects can negate any positive gains in cognition. Objectively, these treatments don't appear to address all of the factors responsible for AD. If so, then they'd work. Realistically, we need to return to the list of symptoms associated with the disease. Here is a list for your perusal:

- Memory dysfunction
- Frontal lobe issues such as problems with planning, initiation, and problem-solving
- Confusion
- Language and communication disturbances
- Mood disturbances
- Sleep disturbances

Now, this list doesn't seem too long. The problem is that there are at least a dozen factors and/or disorders associated with each of these symptoms. It's just not a reality to think that one thing will cause every dysfunction <u>and</u> disturbance. Therefore, there is not and will never be a 'magic bullet' solution to this problem. If someone tells you such, please refer them to the Stanley's Snake Oil controversy of 1917.[20]

Individuality matters

In the 1950's, a biochemist named Roger Williams wrote a book called Biochemical Individuality. In it, he described biochemical and genetic variations inherent in each person. These variations extended all the way to identical twins. For instance, in complete blood counts(CBCs), it was not uncommon to find variations of up to 10-15% per person, depending upon the parameter.[21] Their normal was not everyone else's normal, and these variations rendered some people more susceptible to disease and dysfunction than others. Couple this with the fact that not everyone is exposed to the same factors contributing to disease and dysfunction, it is easy to see that we are looking at many inputs to the disease process. One solution will not address every factor or variation in factors. Please keep this in mind.

Why genetics aren't responsible in most cases

According to most studies on Alzheimer's Disease, genetics account for only 3-4% of all Alzheimer cases worldwide. The most prominent genetic deterministic factors are three autosomal dominant genes for early-onset Alzheimer's Disease (EOAD). They are the presenilin 1 (PSEN1), presenilin 2 (PSEN2), and the amyloid precursor protein (APP). Apolipoprotein E e4 is a fourth gene which renders susceptibility to late-onset Alzheimer's Disease (LOAD).[22] This means that 96-97% of Alzheimer cases are sporadic, meaning no known cause. But we run into a definition problem. People interpret the words 'no known cause' into 'we don't know the cause but there must be **one**'. Sadly, this is the mistake that has led to a slow but steady increase in the number of Alzheimer cases.

5

Why pharmaceuticals are an unlikely successful treatment

Clinical trials

In 2021 alone, the Alzheimer Drug Discovery Foundation identified 208 active clinical trials utilizing drugs with disease modifying action.[23] Multiply this by several decades and you can see why the pharmaceutical approach is not as promising as one would hope. Still, researchers are working around the clock in search of something with benefit.

Anecdotal evidences for better success with alternative treatment

There have been reports by Dr. Mary Newport and others about the reversal of their loved one's Alzheimer's related dementia through the use of up to 4-6 tablespoons of coconut oil.[24] The medium chain triglycerides (MCTs) found in coconut oil are metabolized into ketone bodies, which the brain can utilize as an alternative source of energy. In addition, the monolauric acid found in it has antimicrobial properties. These agents are not utilized in most clinical trials. However, where there is smoke, there is fire. Cerecin Neurosciences introduced a product in 2009 called Axona. Its therapeutic component is one of coconut oil's MCTs called caprylic acid. While the FDA has not approved Axona as a drug to treat Alzheimer's Disease, the product has been generally recognized as safe (GRAS).[25] Cerecin also conducted a Phase II clinical trial which demonstrated a significant cognitive score as compared to a placebo.[26]

6

Prevention and Recovery

I **was told that there is nothing I can do**

"There is no cure for Alzheimer's Disease". We've heard this over and over again. "Try stimulating your brain with crossword puzzles or the like". "Exercise a bit". That's about it, Joe. Let's re-define the statement, shall we? "There is no magic bullet for Alzheimer's Disease". In other words, there is not a single treatment for Alzheimer's Disease. That's true! However, there is a terrific protocol called ReCODE that was introduced by Dr. Dale Bredesen (UCLA) in 2014. It identifies 36+ metabolic imbalances contributing to Alzheimer's Disease and addresses as many of them as possible.[27] The preclinical and clinical success rates of reversal of cognitive decline hover around 75-80%. This is remarkable. So, there is something that you can do. Unfortunately, this intervention is not usually covered by medical insurance; so, you'll have to intervene on behalf of yourself or your loved ones.

I know you're asking the question of why you don't know about this protocol. Let's be honest. The professional community rarely speaks about it. All you hear about is the latest clinical trial with promising results for the treatment of AD. Heck, you don't even hear when these trials are halted due to side effects like encephalitis. What do you expect? Maybe it's time to stop listening to marketing about the latest and greatest trial and start investigating treatments that currently work, along with their cognitive score data and testimonies.

Simplicity

The ReCODE protocol is simple in concept but not in execution. Identify as many factors contributing to AD and then re-balance them to produce a reversal of cognitive decline. I like the word 'simplicity', though. Isn't it refreshingly simple to embrace the concept that a myriad of identifiable factors(which are reversible) contributed to disease rather than hold onto the fear of 'we don't know'?

The possibilities are real

Dr. Bredesen, and now others, have published similar protocols. You can find their papers and results on Pubmed and in books submitted by other publishers. This is not the time to sit and ruminate on the possibilities in the future. The realities are here...today. Embrace them. For too long, we've sat in the dark on issues relevant to our health. And while I don't see a complete paradigm shift for another 50 years, I truly believe that we are close to an explosion of great health for those that are tired of the same old rant about 'the cure'.

You can't go it alone

All you have to do is look at one research paper on the ReCODE protocol to see that it takes trained experts to guide one through the recovery process. The 2014 paper shared many of the identifiable factors that needed addressing[29]:

- Heavy metal toxicity – chelation therapy may be necessary
- Medium chain triglycerides – may need as a source of energy for brain function
- Focus – increased through the use of pantothenic acid (vitamin B5)
- Optimizing the mitochondrial – may need to incorporate the antioxidant Coenzyme Q10 (CoQ10) and other factors
- Treat sleep apnea
- Optimizing zinc to copper ratios
- Optimizing use of the vitamin E complex
- Providing structural components of the synapse – through the use of docosahexaenoic acid (DHA; an omega-3 fatty acid)
- Increasing nerve growth factor – using substances like acetyl-L-carnitine (amino acid)
- Optimizing vitamin D levels – this will vary genetically, depending upon your ethnicity
- Utilizing substances that reduce beta-amyloid load – curcumin and ashwagandha are ideal
- Restoring gastrointestinal health – via probiotics, prebiotics, and other substances
- Balancing hormones – this is especially important since women are more susceptible to AD than men (over 60%)[28]

- Reducing fasting insulin levels - omega-3 fatty acids may play an important role
- Increasing vitamin B12 levels
- Reducing homocysteine levels - achieved through the use of the vitamin B complex
- Brain stimulation and exercise
- Optimizing sleep - there is a reason we've been told to get 8 hours of sleep!
- Reducing stress - stress can affect nearly every physiological parameter in the body
- Optimizing diet - goal is to reduce overall inflammation

As you can see, this is not so easy to do. You must invest in relevant blood work, therapies, and supplements. A single physician can optimize all of these parameters for you. It takes a team of specialists working together. It also takes time. Undoubtedly, you're looking at 6-12 months of working on the majority of these areas. But in the end, if you're in the beginning to middle stages of Alzheimer's Disease, reversal of dementia is possible.

7

You must understand that lifestyle choices are paramount

Convenience, the contemporary path to destruction

Life is fast-paced these days. You've got your job. Instant gratification tools (cell phones, computers, TV) are abundant and being used. You may have children. The house or apartment needs tending, if you're not the messy type. You need to sleep. You need to eat. Oh wait...eating. Your idea is to get something convenient. "Hey, I'll just go to my neighborhood fast food joints for breakfast, lunch, and dinner." "Hey, my kids eat these pre-packaged lunch-thingys. Maybe I can eat them, too. I can get them at my grocery store at 10 for $10. Does the Starving Guy TV dinner still exist?"

People are waking up to the reality that these quick-to-go meals are not nutritionally sound. Even worse, they are usually processed with excessively high amounts omega-6 fatty acids (e.g., linoleic acid) which can massively increase body inflammation and reduce insulin signaling.[30]

However, using the ReCODE protocol as an example, aren't we supposed to be reducing body inflammation and increasing insulin sensitivity? Exactly.

One moment. Aren't you forgetting the electromagnetic frequencies coming from our instant gratification devices? Aren't they supposed to be harmful, and don't they contribute to suboptimal health. The short answer is 'possibly'. I'll address this in another book.

The correct definition of health and pursuing it

Let's examine the World Health Organization's (WHO) definition of health:

"Health is a state of complete physical, mental, and social well-being and not merely the absence of disease or infirmity."

Looking at this statement critically, you can infer how physical health contributes to the other two forms of health. Simply look at a person who has failing physical health with accompanying high levels of chronic pain. That person may be moody or even angry much of the time. They may be quick to snap at you or their caretakers. Why? Pain creates character distortion. Patients may come off as having mental disturbances. People may not want to be around them because of their social ineptitude.

I don't have a problem with the WHO's definition of health. We just need to pursue it, intelligibly. Increased stress, poor sleep, poor nutrition, etc. all need to be brought under control. Please don't complain about having to achieve these goals. They are a must. When you do them, your fears of developing Alzheimer's Disease become markedly reduced as your physiological parameters improve. Just seek them.

8

Identifying toxins and removing their sources

Identifying toxins in the body typically involves a combination of medical history, physical examination, and specific blood tests or other laboratory investigations. The choice of blood tests depends on the suspected toxins and their potential effects on the body. Here are some common blood tests that may be used to identify toxins:

- **Complete Blood Count (CBC)** - Changes in these counts can sometimes indicate exposure to toxins or the presence of certain types of toxins, such as heavy metals.
- **Liver Function Tests (LFTs)** - Liver function tests assess the health and function of the liver by measuring levels of enzymes and other substances in the blood. Elevated levels of liver enzymes, such as alanine aminotransferase (ALT) and aspartate aminotransferase (AST), may indicate liver damage due to toxin exposure, such as alcohol or certain medications.
- **Renal Function Tests** - These tests evaluate kidney function

by measuring levels of substances such as creatinine and blood urea nitrogen (BUN) in the blood. Kidneys play a crucial role in filtering toxins from the blood, so abnormalities in renal function tests may indicate kidney damage or dysfunction due to toxin exposure.
- **Toxicology Screen** - A toxicology screen is a comprehensive test that can detect the presence of various drugs and toxins in the blood. It may include tests for substances such as illicit drugs, prescription medications, alcohol, and certain chemicals or toxins.
- **Heavy Metal Testing** - Specific blood tests can measure levels of heavy metals, such as lead, mercury, arsenic, and cadmium, which can accumulate in the body and cause toxicity over time. These tests typically require specialized analysis and may not be part of routine laboratory testing.
- **Environmental Exposure Tests** - In cases of suspected environmental toxin exposure, such as pesticides or industrial chemicals, blood tests may be used to measure levels of specific toxins or their metabolites in the blood. These tests can help assess the extent of exposure and guide treatment decisions.

Interpretation alone is a reason that you cannot, as previously mentioned, 'go it alone'. Blood test results require careful consideration of individual factors, including symptoms, medical history, and potential sources of toxin exposure. Additionally, other diagnostic tests or imaging studies may be necessary to confirm toxin exposure and assess its effects on the body. Consulting with trained professionals is essential for proper evaluation and management of toxin exposure.

Do protocols to remove toxins exist? What do the medical and scientific literature say about their validity?

Protocols to remove toxins from the body exist and are commonly referred to as detoxification or detox protocols. These protocols aim to support the body's natural detoxification processes and may involve lifestyle changes, dietary modifications, supplementation, and other therapeutic interventions such as chelation.

It's important to note that the effectiveness and safety of detox protocols can vary widely; however, none of these approaches lack scientific evidence...not even chelation.

Some common components of detox protocols include:

- **Dietary Changes** - Many detox protocols emphasize consuming whole, nutrient-dense foods and avoiding processed foods, sugar, caffeine, alcohol, and other potentially harmful substances. Certain foods and beverages, such as fruits, vegetables, herbal teas, and water with lemon, may be promoted for their purported detoxifying effects.
- **Hydration** - Adequate hydration is essential for supporting the body's natural detoxification processes. Drinking plenty of water helps flush toxins from the body through urine and sweat.
- **Supplements** - Some detox protocols include the use of dietary supplements, such as vitamins, minerals, antioxidants, and herbs, to support detoxification pathways and enhance liver function. Common supplements used in detox protocols may include milk thistle, N-acetylcysteine (NAC),

glutathione, and activated charcoal, among others.
- **Exercise** - Regular physical activity can support detoxification by promoting circulation, sweating, and lymphatic drainage. Exercise also helps reduce stress and inflammation, which are important considerations in detoxification.
- **Sauna Therapy** - Sweating induced by sauna therapy is believed to help eliminate toxins from the body through the skin. Skin is one of the back-up organs for elimination. Sauna sessions may be included as part of detox protocols, although evidence supporting their effectiveness for detoxification is limited.
- **Stress Reduction** - Chronic stress can impair detoxification processes and contribute to toxin accumulation in the body. Stress reduction techniques such as meditation, deep breathing exercises, yoga, and massage therapy may be recommended as part of detox protocols.
- **Chelation Therapy** - The word "chelation" is derived from the Greek word "chele," meaning claw. It refers to the way chelating agents bind to metal ions or other toxins and form stable, water-soluble complexes that can be excreted from the body via the kidneys.

At this point, you may be thinking that you can do this all by yourself. Think again. Overburdening the bloodstream with too many toxins often results in a Herxheimer reaction or a healing detoxification reaction. Herxheimer reactions are bodily responses to microbial die-off while healing detoxifications are the result of an excess of toxins. Neither are pleasant, unless being nauseated and having migraines are your thing.

Move?

Do you live near a factory, processing plant, or other industrial facility that is spewing waste into the immediate air that you breathe? Do you know of situations where many people living in close proximity to these facilities have developed cancers, Alzheimer's, and other maladies? Are you one of those people? Well then, please consider moving. What, relocating? YES! Detoxification of bodily systems can be extensive and may involve persistence over long periods of time. This is usually because of high amounts of toxins embedded into tissue due to prolonged periods of time. Moving to a cleaner environment can help speed up the detoxification process by minimizing exposure.

Who can I trust to guide me along this path?

This is a no-brainer. An established practitioner with a long track record of both successes and an ability to navigate through the nuances of the protocol. (Remember: everyone is biochemically and genetically distinct). Don't mess around. Be diligent and do your homework on who is qualified to perform such tasks.

9

Mindset

Y*oung adults – why you should spend the money now to stay healthy*

Excellent health is hard work! Let me explain. You don't have to stay in the gym for 6 hours per day to achieve great health. In fact, you may want to stay out of the gym for such an extended time because of the time constraints and additional physiological stressors on the body from the exercise. Also, ideally, you want to minimize consumption of processed food. This will cost money. We all know that eating grass-fed meat and organic produce isn't cheap. However, these will help establish and prolong excellent health as you age. Lastly, setting up a place of residence where toxins are minimized, outside of the woods, is probably going to be costly. (Please refer to low-income inner city residents who are stuck with living next to garbage incinerators, bus station and repair facilities, or other toxin spewers, if you have questions or comments.) If the 'why?' isn't obvious, then contemplate the fact that 60% of people that go bankrupt in this country do so because of medical expenses;

and over 70% of them had medical insurance. Spend the money now to stay healthy because medical expenses are a pain to cover. It'll be far cheaper in the long run, if you do.

Elderly years – why you should spend the money now, as well!

Hi folks, you don't have the luxury to sit around and wait. Time is precious and so is quality of life. Spend your remaining years in good health. This may involve getting healthy first. So be it. Get healthy and then stay healthy by spending the money to achieve it the correct way.

Roadblocks to achieving your best health

Common roadblocks are:

- Fear of stepping outside of what you've heard on mainstream media
- Fear of the unknown
- The cost of a truly healthy lifestyle
- Fear...
- Fear...
- Fear...

(no, I'm not being sarcastic)

Don't be afraid.

10

Conclusions

Alright, I've tried to walk you through the critical thinking that you should possess when considering chronic diseases like Alzheimer's. It's not so scary. Indeed, pausing to dutifully consider things through eases fears and enlightens both you and those around you on the realities of the situation. Embrace your health...I'm rooting for you!

If you found this book helpful, I'd be appreciative if you left a favorable review for this publication on Amazon!

11

Resources

1. Hippius H, Neundörfer G. The discovery of Alzheimer's disease. (2003). *Dialogues Clin Neurosci.*, 5(1), 101–108. https://doi.org/10.31887/DCNS.2003.5.1/hhippius
2. Lucci, B. The contribution of Gaetano Perusini to the definition of Alzheimer's disease. (1998). *Ital J Neuro Sci 19*, 49–52. https://doi.org/10.1007/BF03028813
3. Smith, T. L. (1908). [Review of *Rivista Italiana di Neuropatologia, Psichiatria ed Elettroterapia*]. *The American Journal of Psychology*, 19(3), 425–426. https://doi.org/10.2307/1413212
4. *The Neuropathological Hallmarks of Alzheimer's Disease.* (2021, August 24). https://altoida.com/blog/the-neuropathological-hallmarks-of-alzheimers-disease/
5. Haass, C., Kaether, C., Thinakaran, G., & Sisodia, S. (2012). Trafficking and proteolytic processing of APP. *Cold Spring Harbor perspectives in medicine*, 2(5), a006270. https://doi.org/10.1101/cshperspect.a006270
6. Suh, Y. H., & Checler, F. (2002). Amyloid precursor protein,

presenilins, and alpha-synuclein: molecular pathogenesis and pharmacological applications in Alzheimer's disease. *Pharmacological reviews*, 54(3), 469–525. https://doi.org/10.1124/pr.54.3.469

7. Dickson, T. C., & Vickers, J. C. (2001). The morphological phenotype of beta-amyloid plaques and associated neuritic changes in Alzheimer's disease. *Neuroscience*, 105(1), 99–107. https://doi.org/10.1016/s0306-4522(01)00169-5

8. Tsering, W., & Prokop, S. (2024). Neuritic Plaques - Gateways to Understanding Alzheimer's Disease. *Molecular neurobiology*, 61(5), 2808–2821. https://doi.org/10.1007/s12035-023-03736-7

9. Alonso, A. C., Li, B., Grundke-Iqbal, I., & Iqbal, K. (2008). Mechanism of tau-induced neurodegeneration in Alzheimer disease and related tauopathies. *Current Alzheimer research*, 5(4), 375–384. https://doi.org/10.2174/156720508785132307

10. Kidd M. (1963). Paired helical filaments in electron microscopy of Alzheimer's disease. *Nature*, 197, 192–193. https://doi.org/10.1038/197192b0

11. Kril, J. J., Patel, S., Harding, A. J., & Halliday, G. M. (2002). Neuron loss from the hippocampus of Alzheimer's disease exceeds extracellular neurofibrillary tangle formation. *Acta neuropathologica*, 103(4), 370–376. https://doi.org/10.1007/s00401-001-0477-5

12. Tagarelli, A., Piro, A., Tagarelli, G., Lagonia, P., & Quattrone, A. (2006). Alois Alzheimer: a hundred years after the discovery of the eponymous disorder. *International journal of biomedical science : IJBS*, 2(2), 196–204.

13. Krstic, D., & Knuesel, I. (2013). Deciphering the mechanism

underlying late-onset Alzheimer disease. *Nature reviews. Neurology, 9*(1), 25–34. https://doi.org/10.1038/nrneurol.2012.236

14. Yang, Z., Zou, Y., & Wang, L. (2023). Neurotransmitters in Prevention and Treatment of Alzheimer's Disease. *International journal of molecular sciences, 24*(4), 3841. https://doi.org/10.3390/ijms24043841

15. Bakulski, K. M., Seo, Y. A., Hickman, R. C., Brandt, D., Vadari, H. S., Hu, H., & Park, S. K. (2020). Heavy Metals Exposure and Alzheimer's Disease and Related Dementias. *Journal of Alzheimer's disease : JAD, 76*(4), 1215–1242. https://doi.org/10.3233/JAD-200282

16. Das, N., Raymick, J., & Sarkar, S. (2021). Role of metals in Alzheimer's disease. *Metabolic brain disease, 36*(7), 1627–1639. https://doi.org/10.1007/s11011-021-00765-w

17. Kao, Y. C., Ho, P. C., Tu, Y. K., Jou, I. M., & Tsai, K. J. (2020). Lipids and Alzheimer's Disease. *International journal of molecular sciences, 21*(4), 1505. https://doi.org/10.3390/ijms21041505

18. Xu Lou, I., Ali, K., & Chen, Q. (2023). Effect of nutrition in Alzheimer's disease: A systematic review. *Frontiers in neuroscience, 17*, 1147177. https://doi.org/10.3389/fnins.2023.1147177

19. Breijyeh, Z., & Karaman, R. (2020). Comprehensive Review on Alzheimer's Disease: Causes and Treatment. *Molecules (Basel, Switzerland), 25*(24), 5789. https://doi.org/10.3390/molecules25245789

20. *Snake oil.* (n.d.). Retrieved June 1, 2024, from https://en.wikipedia.org/wiki/Snake_oil

21. Williams, R. (1956). *Biochemical Individuality.* McGraw Hill Professional.

22. Williamson, J., Goldman, J., & Marder, K. S. (2009). Genetic aspects of Alzheimer disease. *The neurologist*, 15(2), 80–86. https://doi.org/10.1097/NRL.0b013e318187e76b
23. Fillit, H. & Alzheimer's Drug Discovery Foundation. (2021). *ALZHEIMER'S CLINICAL TRIALS REPORT.*
24. *Steve's Story: Dr. Mary Newport's personal triumph over early onset.* (2018, July 14). Foundation for Alternative and Integrative Medicine. https://www.faim.org/steves-story-dr-mary-newports-personal-triumph-over-early-onset-alzheimers
25. *Axona.* (n.d.) Wikipedia. Retrieved June 1, 2024, from https://en.wikipedia.org/wiki/Axona
26. Henderson, S. T., Vogel, J. L., Barr, L. J., Garvin, F., Jones, J. J., & Costantini, L. C. (2009). Study of the ketogenic agent AC-1202 in mild to moderate Alzheimer's disease: a randomized, double-blind, placebo-controlled, multicenter trial. *Nutrition & metabolism*, 6, 31. https://doi.org/10.1186/1743-7075-6-31
27. Manager. (2023, March 16). *Bredesen protocol.* Apollo Health. https://www.apollohealthco.com/bredesen-protocol/
28. Mielke M. M. (2018). Sex and Gender Differences in Alzheimer's Disease Dementia. *The Psychiatric times*, 35(11), 14–17.
29. Bredesen, D. E., Amos, E. C., Canick, J., Ackerley, M., Raji, C., Fiala, M., & Ahdidan, J. (2016). Reversal of cognitive decline in Alzheimer's disease. *Aging*, 8(6), 1250–1258. https://doi.org/10.18632/aging.100981
30. Mamounis, K. J., Yasrebi, A., & Roepke, T. A. (2017). Linoleic acid causes greater weight gain than saturated fat without hypothalamic inflammation in the male mouse. *The Journal*

of nutritional biochemistry, *40*, 122–131. https://doi.org/10.1016/j.jnutbio.2016.10.016

www.ingramcontent.com/pod-product-compliance
Lightning Source LLC
Chambersburg PA
CBHW050249230526
45470CB00005B/2178